Love Your

Liver

Lose Weight &
Beat Food & Alcohol
Addiction

David Ash B.Sc. Nutrition

David Ash

2013

British Library Cataloguing–in-Publication Data
ISBN 978-0-9550857-6-5

*"The problem we are faced with is people eat for
palatability not nutrition."* John Yudkin (lecture)

*The word 'Liver' comes from the word
'Live'. Care of the liver is the key to
health and a long and happy life.*

This book is a private health publication
Sponsored by Joy Doreen Ash

NHS Statistics for 2012

In 2008 Alcohol cost the NHS

£2.8 Billion

- **6,669 alcohol deaths** in 2010 – 22% up on 2001

- **4,275 (64%) died from alcohol liver disease**

- **813,600 hospital admissions caused by alcohol**

- **198,900 (24%) of these due to alcohol consumption**

- 167,764 prescriptions for alcohol dependency in 2011 cost

£2.49 million

Drug abuse expert Dr. Sidney Cohen, described **alcohol** as

"the most dangerous drug on earth"

If ALCOHOL is the most dangerous drug on earth, WHY IS IT ON SALE EVERYWHERE?

Stupid question: Experts agree that alcohol is more dangerous than ecstasy (See BBC Horizon) and ecstasy is classified as a Class A drug so why isn't alcohol classified as a Class A drug?

Alcohol, THE LEGAL DRUG is the FIFTH CAUSE OF DEATH

But there is a drug more deadly than alcohol.

It is *the* top killer and *the* least regulated!

SUGAR!

let's be clear what sugar is!

As far as your body is concerned sugar is
GLUCOSE. What we usually call sugar is
SUCROSE which is only half GLUCOSE.
Starch in potatoes, bread, etc. is

100% GLUCOSE

You may call it starch but to your body
starch is sugar. Sugar is glucose and
glucose is essential to life. If you cut off
the supply of glucose to your brain you
would first go into a coma and then die.

- ❖ **Too little sugar will kill you.**
- ❖ **The right amount of sugar is essential for life & health.**
- ❖ **Too much sugar will kill you.**

Sugar = Energy
Energy is stored as Fat

Sugar is also stored in the liver as glycogen.

When sugar levels rise in the blood the body secretes **INSULIN**. Insulin causes blood sugar ~ glucose ~ to be converted into glycogen and fat. As blood sugar levels fall we get the sugar blues. Craving for sugar, we head for the biscuit tin, the sticky bun, the chocolate bar or another slice of bread and jam. These spike insulin levels and set off the craving all over again. This is the cycle of carbohydrate

ADDICTION
Most affluent people suffer from
CARBOHYDRATE ADDICTION
Most of us are sugar junkies

SUGAR IS ADDICTIVE
FOOD INDUSTRY IS A
LEGAL DRUG TRADE

Eating excessive sugar due to carbohydrate addiction leads to the build up of **fat in the liver,** fat around the vital organs and **fat in the arteries** ~ CHOLESTEROL.

Being fat is not a problem. Fat spread over a body can be beautiful and healthy but **BELLY FAT** is a warning of metabolic syndrome ~ the onset of diabetes, obesity & circulatory disease caused by **fat in the arteries** which is...**The Number One** cause of **DEATH** in the affluent nations as it leads to circulatory diseases including:
HIGH BLOOD PRESSURE
HEART ATTACKS
STROKE

The fat is in our arteries not because we eat too much fat...

...but because we eat too much **SUGAR** in confectionary, cake, biscuits, syrup, cereals, chocolate and **STARCH** in crisps, corn, bread, potatoes, pasta, crackers, & white rice.

& BREAD IS BAD

Bread is starch & gluten
- put that way it sounds OK but -

Gluten is a gluey protein that damages the small intestine causing celiac disease. It literally glues up our guts. While most people don't have celiac disease many are 'wheat sensitive' and feel bloated and heavy after eating bread ~ especially fresh doughy bread ~ you know the 'healthy' brown stuff with phytate in the fibre that locks calcium, magnesium and other essential minerals...

...not to mention yeast that exacerbates

Candida

The Staff of life?
Give us a break!

BREAD

and cake are

SUGAR

& GUT

GLUE

The exception is baked beans on toast. The amino acids in gluten compliment those in beans to make an inexpensive equivalent to good quality protein.

IT'S NOT THEY ARE ADDING SUGAR TO PRACTICALLY EVERYTHING; PRACTICALLY EVERYTHING IS SUGAR!

In a supermarket, to see the real extent shelves are stacked with the addictive drug sugar in bright cartons packaged as any number of delicious foods...

...all you have to do is scratch the word *starch* and replace it with the word *sugar*...

...and the stuff we call sugar (sucrose) is in practically everything anyway, including a number of brands in legal

ROWS OF THE OTHER DRUG ~ ALCOHOL...

...and near the pampered towers of vitamin enriched toilet paper you may spot a few shelves of eggs blamed for heart disease because they contain cholesterol. That is...

The Great Fat Scam

It was 1971. I was a first year student in the nutrition department of Queen Elizabeth College of London University and John Yudkin, (author of *Pure White and Deadly*) was my professor ~ In 1957 Dr Yudkin was the pioneer who had first proclaimed sugar as a cause of heart disease because it raises the levels of insulin in the blood.

I remember the incident to this day. I was standing with a group of about six students when John Yudkin walked by. One of the students questioned him about the popular misconception that dietary fat causes heart disease. The professor rose up and declared: *"There is no evidence of a link between dietary fat and heart disease, there never was and there never will be!"*

This is not to say all fat is good for you. Fat is very rich in calories and they will make you fat. We are told saturated fat is not good and the hydrogenated fat added to processed food is down right bad for us. But I recall in my childhood how we were told by misguided parents to spread synthetic slime full of dangerous trans-fatty acids on bread which should have been enjoyed with golden butter blessed with essential fatty acids. Who told us that margarine is better than butter ~ **CORPORATE DRUG BARONS OF FOOD INDUSTRY OF COURSE!** Their strategy was to blame heart disease on butter and cream, milk and eggs. Point the finger at the beleaguered farmers growing natural food. Ignore the fact people have been eating eggs, butter and cream for thousands of years without heart disease. Spread the spin to build the market for all the new post war products of the burgeoning food industry. Ensure universities and the media back the corporate story through generous research grants and advertising revenue.

That is how to pull off a great fat

SCAM

This is how they did it. During the Korean War the American MASH carried out autopsies on Korean soldiers as well as US GIs. Fatty streaks in the arteries of the US troops characteristic of the onset of circulatory disease were absent in the arteries of the Koreans. US scientists proclaimed the only difference between the Americans and Koreans was their fat intake. They concluded, conveniently, that dietary fat was the cause of heart disease. They forgot to mention that **Americans eat enormous plates of processed food whereas the Asians ate small portions of natural food.**

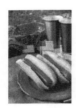 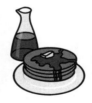 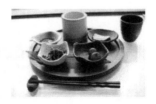

The experts overlooked through stupidity or ignored through cupidity the difference in the sugar and calorie intake of war torn half starved Koreans and well fed American service men...

THE RESEARCH from

the Harvard School of Public Health website: The low-fat, high-starch diet that was the focus of dietary advice during the 1990s-as reflected by the USDA food guide pyramid-is dying out. A growing body of evidence has been pointing to its inadequacy for weight loss or prevention of heart disease and several cancers. The final nail in the coffin comes from an eight-year trial that included almost 49,000 women.

The trial and its findings

The Women's Health Initiative Dietary Modification Trial was started back in 1993, at a time when dietary fat was seen as a dietary evil and the low-fat diet was thought to be a straightforward route to preventing heart disease, some cancers, and the epidemic of obesity that was beginning to sweep the country. With funding from the National Heart, Lung, and Blood Institute, researchers recruited almost 50,000 women between the ages of 50 and 79 years. Of these, 19,541 were randomly assigned to follow a low-fat diet. Their goal was to lower their fat intake from almost 38% of calories to 20%. They were helped in this effort by a series of individual and group counseling sessions. Another 29,294 women were randomly assigned to continue their usual diets, and were given just generic diet-related educational materials. After eight years, the researchers looked at how many (and what percentage) of women in each group had developed breast cancer or colorectal cancer. They tallied up heart attacks, strokes, and other forms of heart disease. They also looked at things like weight gain or loss, cholesterol levels, and other measures of health. **The results, published in the *Journal of the American Medical Association*, showed no benefits for a low-fat diet.** Women assigned to this eating strategy did not appear to gain protection against breast cancer, colorectal cancer, or cardiovascular disease. After eight years, their weights were generally the same as those of women following their usual diets...the WHI trial was, by far, the most expensive study of diet ever conducted (costing many hundreds of millions of dollars)... the women in the low-fat group received intensive dietary counseling from some of the best nutritionists and dietitians in the country....

References

1. Prentice RL, Caan B, Chlebowski RT, et al. Low-fat dietary pattern and risk of invasive breast cancer: the Women's Health Initiative Randomized Controlled Dietary Modification Trial. JAMA. 2006; 295:629-42.
2. Beresford SA, Johnson KC, Ritenbaugh C, et al. Low-fat dietary pattern and risk of colorectal cancer: the Women's Health Initiative Randomized Controlled Dietary Modification Trial. JAMA. 2006; 295:643-54.
3. Howard BV, Van Horn L, Hsia J, et al. Low-fat dietary pattern and risk of cardiovascular disease: the Women's Health Initiative Randomized Controlled Dietary Modification Trial. JAMA. 2006; 295:655-66.
4. Howard BV, Manson JE, Stefanick ML, et al. Low-fat dietary pattern and weight change over 7 years: the Women's Health Initiative Dietary Modification Trial. JAMA. 2006; 295:39-49.

Driven by the Great American Dream – some might call it the **Great Pursuit of Gain** - few had listened to that irritating fellow Yudkin threatening the refined carbohydrate drug cartel. In South America they would have shot him. In the North they just ignored him!

In 1972, John Yudkin had published his book linking gun running and slavery to sugar. Like the drugs cocaine and heroin, sugar has a history of violence and enslavement, cruelty and greed. The guns may have gone but the greed continues unabated and with it all the diseases suffered by the unfortunate addicts.

So what can we do?

Protest

Forget it!

THERE IS TOO MUCH MONEY IN THE LICENSED DRUG TRADES INCLUDING

MEDICAL DRUGS

Medical Drugs are a massive money spinner and like any other drug they can be absolutely deadly

Adverse Prescribed Drug Reactions hospitalized 2.2 million people in the US in a year of which 106,000 died, "making these reactions between the fourth and sixth leading cause of death."* *Journal of American Medical Association (JAMA)* 4-15-**1998**

"From 1998 through 2005, reported serious adverse drug events increased 2.6-fold and fatal adverse drug events increased 2.7-fold..." *Archives of Internal Medicine,* p 1752, Sep 10, 2007

The World Health Organisation states online:

- Unintended, harmful reactions to medicines (known as adverse drug reactions) are among the leading causes of death in many countries.*
- The majority of adverse drug reactions (ADR) are preventable.
- People in every country are affected by ADRs.
- In some countries ADR-related costs, such as hospitalization, surgery and lost productivity, exceed the cost of the medications.

Stupid Question: *Why aren't deaths due to prescribed drugs included in the UK official published causes of death?*

THERE IS A TERRIBLE TIME BOMB TICKING...

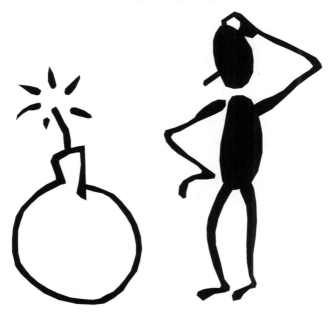

THE BABY BOOMER GENERATION OF FOOD & ALCOHOL ADDICTS IS GROWING OLDER AND SICKER.

- OBESITY IS EPIDEMIC
- DIABETES IS EPIDEMIC
- ALCOHOL RELATED LIVER DISEASE IS EPIDEMIC

The NHS is reaching breaking point as the baby boomers come to the age when many will spend their last years of long lingering life in pension poverty, alcohol, sugar & supermarket food dependency and chronic ill health: RETIREMENT...

...and who will pay for their care?

Question: What can I do about the corporate drug trades that are robbing me of my health?

Answer: I can take responsibility for my own health. I can resort to education before medication. I can choose what I put in my mouth.

Question: How can I ensure that when I reach retirement age I will be healthy enough to enjoy the freedom and the well earned fruits of my labours?

Answer: Read on and all will be revealed!

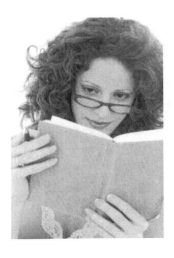

I have been seeking the secret to good **health through nutrition** for 50 years. I started work with my Dad replacing minerals in refined sugar at age 16 and at 18, I was apprentice to his sorcery formulating a vitamin C, charcoal and kaolin concoction to deal with alcohol. Convinced that the nutritionists of today would be the doctors of tomorrow I studied nutrition rather than medicine and went on to try macrobiotic & vegetarian, then vegan, fruitarian & raw food diets. I even lived on light for a month but I had a natural aversion to life long restrictions. While some may do, I didn't thrive on restrictive diets: usually rich in carbohydrates. I thrive on an evening meal of steamed vegetables and fish or nut cutlets, bean burgers and meat once or twice a week. I have always taken supplements, especially antioxidants, minerals and phytonutrients, but I never felt 100% after lunch. The problem was energy. I felt lethargic after eating in the day and needed siestas and cat naps. I was eating too many carbs in the day ~ cereal and bread, crackers and biscuits. Despite my knowledge I was still a sugar junkie. There was something missing. I knew my health was still in danger.

Then one evening I saw the light...

...it came out of the television set...

I had a revelation...

...through a BBC TV Horizon Programme...

I was educated by my mum...

...she chose the channel.

Thank God for Mum and the BBC despite Jimmy Savile

Amen

I was staying with my 92 year old mother. She announced we were going to watch a programme on fasting on BBC2. Peering up from the TV pages in her *Western Morning News* Ma said it sounded very interesting, right up my street as a nutritionist. I thought it sounded like a return to lent and monastic life. I loved my food and hated fasting. I did it on Good Friday once a decade maybe but being one not to argue with Ma, when the hour with *Horizon* finally arrived, I settled on the sofa and proceeded to watch. In years I had never been so impacted by an evening of television. On Wed the 5th September 2012 I was mesmerized. Michael Mosley appeared to have discovered the Holy Grail of Health; how to live a long and healthy life, stay young and lose weight with minimal lifestyle changes. As the programme unfolded the new science behind the ancient idea of fasting revealed we can fast and still enjoy our food. Michael was testing out the science of fasting on himself - with life-changing results. I looked across the room at my mother. She was living proof that what Michael Mosley was saying was true.

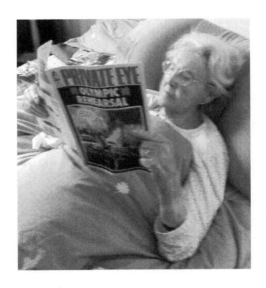

As long as I can remember my mum has fasted and eaten sparingly. She is healthy and sprightly in her nineties. She has a pacemaker and her only medication is a single tablet that goes with it. She is not overweight and is fully *compos mentis*. She can discuss with me politics, physics and philosophy. By the end of one evening of mental gymnastics she even managed to get to grips with:

Heisenberg's Uncertainty Principle!

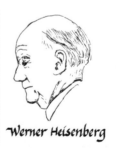

Werner Heisenberg

Michael Mosley had visited a number of universities in the United States where new evidence was presented that people who fast or live on low calorie diets are healthier and live longer than people who eat normally. One scientist said they appeared almost as members of a different species. **Significantly:**

The rates of cancer, circulatory disease, obesity, Alzheimer's and diabetes along with need for medication were shown to be significantly lower in people who fast than in the normal population.

Researchers at the different universities discovered it didn't seem to matter how people fast, improvements **were the same** and occurred **within months** of commencing the practice.

Mosley concluded from all the fasting practices the easiest to follow was to

Reduce food intake to 600 calories (Kcal) two days a week.

He said he was determined to fast two days a week for the rest of his life. As I watched the programme I was converted, I decided to do the same. **Since Sept 2012 I have cut out bread & cake as staples.** I have them now and again when people serve them for me but I endeavour not to buy bread or sandwiches any more. That has reduced my overall calorie intake and increased my energy in the day.

I still enjoy a biscuit with my morning cup of tea but I have cut out breakfast cereal and toast replacing it with grapefruit or a bowl of porridge or a cooked breakfast once a week. Cereal and bread in the morning set up a cycle of hunger leaving me ravenous by lunch. I used to have a sandwich for lunch or rye crisp bread & cheese but I found I was still drained of energy for physical work. I needed breaks and cat naps. Since I cut down on cake and bread and started fasting I have more energy for work and don't need to sleep or rest in the day like I used to.

I look forward to my fast days by giving myself treats reserved for those days. A nutritious low calorie **Clif Bar** at lunch, with a glass of water on a fast day leaves me with ample energy while satisfying my hunger until supper. A Clif bar ~ ordered online - is half the cost of a round of sandwiches so they save money ~ *I never have more than one a day.*

Celery with peanut butter spread in the gap is another treat for my fast lunch instead of gut gluing sandwiches. I relish a Waldorf salad ~ celery, apple, grapes and walnuts enjoying that on some fast days. Alternatively I prepare rocket or watercress with walnuts and feta cheese or grate carrots with white and red cabbage to enjoy with a French dressing or red onion chopped with a fresh orange, olives, olive oil, sea salt and pepper; that is a delicious treat on a fast day.

My usual supper may be steamed veg or salad, with fish or meat, bean burger or nut cutlet or it may be stir fry and tofu or salad and brown rice with dhal. For sweet I usually have fresh or stewed fruit or prunes with yoghurt or custard, ice cream or cream, followed by coffee and chocolate with a small glass of port. I drink wine rarely and spirits or beer even less. I am a teaholic and enjoy a cup of coffee most days but on a fast day I don't drink coffee and I replace morning tea with herb tea, skip the biscuit and have grapefruit for breakfast. My supper is about half my normal portion and for sweet I have fruit (not banana) and no port, chocolate, cream or ice cream. I don't do a strict count of calories I just reduce my overall intake of food to about a third of what I would normally eat in a day. My rule of thumb is: **If I am hungry then I know my fast is working.**

According to the studies presented on the BBC *Horizon* programme it doesn't seem to matter when you eat or what you eat ~ so long as you eat less. You might prepare your main meal at breakfast or lunch or a number of small meals throughout the day (eating small portions is healthier than eating large ones and do remember to drink lots of water).

One of the studies presented on BBC *Horizon* revealed alternating fast days and feast days to be effective so for every day I fast I enjoy a feast day and on the intervening days I make an effort to reduce my overall intake of calories especially bread, buns and cake and other refined carbohydrates I save the food indulgences for my feast days. Feast days are the days I look forward to when I can enjoy whatever foods and drink I like **within reason**. I usually have a feast day at the weekend. Feast days help me keep sugar foods under control. When my own children were toddlers we controlled their demands for sweets every day by declaring: *'Saturday is sweety day'.* I don't find it easy to fast or resist sugary foods. Days of indulgence to look forward to worked for my family when they were children and work for me as an adult. In my opinion it is unrealistic to expect the population to accept a lifelong prohibition on sugary food and alcohol. After a period of fasting the desire for unhealthy food sometimes falls away and the need to over indulge in food and alcohol can decline naturally; that is ideal. But any effort to control sugar and alcohol intake is better than none. Whatever works for you; go for it! Don't be discouraged if you over eat or have a drink on a fast day. Persevere. Keep doing the best you can and eventually you will succeed in cutting calories & alcohol. On the intervening days I endeavour to eat whole foods i.e. brown rice rather than white and whole potatoes rather than peeled and corn or oat porridge with stewed fruit instead of commercial breakfast cereal. I make a point of having plenty of salad or steamed vegetables and fresh fruit. I control my drinking of alcohol – no more than a unit a day – and if I smoke it's very rare – I go through patches of enjoying roll ups then stop altogether for a year or two. Since writing this book I have to tidied up my act to restrict white rice, peeled potatoes pizza and sandwiches, chocolate bars, fry-ups, burgers, fast food, junk food, sugary breakfast cereals, cream buns, cakes, rice crackers, pop, crisps, sugar-in-my-coffee, and keep fried and fatty foods & refined carbohydrates to a minimum.

NEVER BINGE EAT OR BINGE DRINK.
Binge eating will undo the value of fasting and binge drinking can lead to acute liver poisoning and even death.

BALANCE, WHOLESOME LIVING AND A LIGHT APPROACH TO LIFE ARE KEYS TO ATTAINING HEALTH, HAPPINESS & PEACE

REMEMBER RATIONING?

The UK population was healthiest in World War II

Why?

Food was simple, wholesome and scarce!

People drank alcohol but rarely got really drunk.

Everyone smoked so maybe continual overeating is more harmful than smoking?

With declining yields of food due to climate change

With a growing population requiring ever more food

With economic recession making it harder for families to buy enough food

We cannot afford to keep on killing ourselves with food

Fasting means we eat less so there is more for others to eat...

...and everyone is healthier!

ADDITIONAL IDEAS

- Some people fast one day a week on no food just water.
- Some doctors suggest we cut our food portions by half.
- Restrict your visits to fast food restaurants; homecook instead

CUT CALORIES OVERALL. It is vital we REDUCE THE SIZE OF FOOD PORTIONS

IT IS IMPORTANT THAT WE, THE GOLDEN OLDIES, FAST, EAT LESS & DRINK LESS ALCOHOL.

I am 64 and I don't have the same appetite I had when I was 34. As we grow older our need for food declines yet old habits of twenty fags and three square meals a day, plus elevenses and tea with cake at four, a digestive and cup of tea when we rise and cocoa and a cookie when we retire, not to mention cheese and biscuits, a bar of chocolate, two pints of beer, a glass or two of wine, a sherry & a tot of whiskey and/or gin and tonic, and a packet or two of crisps to fill the gaps in between, die hard. Is it any wonder old folk are so sick they have carrier bags full of drugs?

IF YOU ARE OVER SIXTY AND DON'T WANT TO JOIN THE LIVING DEAD, TAKE CONTROL OF YOUR EATING AND YOUR ALCOHOL DRINKING!

Start Fasting Now
BEFORE IT IS TOO LATE!

As hunter gatherers we evolved to go through periods of famine interspaced with glut.

The liver has evolved to have a rest from food occasionally to detox naturally, clean the blood, clear glycogen and reduce fat. It is common sense! So long as we are not starving, to feel hungry sometimes is healthy. With time I have got use to feeling hungry when I fast. I have to remind myself on fast days that it is good to feel hunger and an empty stomach sometimes.

The real problem is the temptation of food and drink. Surrounded as we are by delicious food and drinks in supermarkets and shops, cafes and kitchen cupboards it is not easy to stop eating; especially when we are hungry.

Fasting is easier said than done! When it comes to drinks it is even harder. **ALCOHOL IS A SERIOUSLY ADDICTIVE DRUG THAT CAN LEAD TO MALNUTRITION AND FATAL LIVER DAMAGE.**

On the 20th February 2012, **Alistair Campbell,** Tony Blair's former spokesman gave an impassioned presentation on **BBC Panorama** of his personal battle with alcohol. Along with alarming statistics of just how serious the problem of alcohol has become since licensing restrictions have been dropped and cheap alcohol has become available on supermarket shelves he drew attention to the danger of wine being added to the national consumption of beer and spirits. On the programme Alistair Campbell also said the government recommends that we abstain from alcohol two days a week...

He was suggesting we only have to abstain from alcohol two days a week. We don't have to give up drinking permanently. We just need to give ourselves a break from the bottle now and again. NO ALCOHOL ON FAST DAYS MAKES SENSE!

THE LIVER NEEDS RECOVERY TIME

If you were to work 24/7 all your life and never had a break it would kill you. **So now you know what is killing you!**

Eating loads of food and drinking a lot of alcohol, without ever giving the liver a break, can lead to an **EARLY GRAVE!**

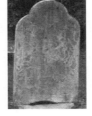

Give Your Liver a Break!

Look after your liver
♥Love your liver♥

JUST TWO DAYS A WEEK

Choose two days in the week that are most convenient. Abstain from alcohol, fags and sugar ~ that includes bread, white rice, peeled potatoes, pasta, cereal, cakes, biscuits, crackers etc and reduce substantially your overall food intake. If you cannot manage 48 hours straight, have a fill day between two fast days. Do what works for you. If you don't manage two days on 600 calories TRY A SINGLE DAY A WEEK FASTING ON WATER ALONE. Stay positive. Do the best you can and take on the challenge. **NEVER GIVE UP!**

Great, now fired and inspired we can go into the pubs with a bell and challenge the locals to fast and stop boozing two days a week to save their livers and the NHS a staggering **£2.8 Billion a year!**

Get real!

Telling people to abstain from alcohol and food will never work unless we take into account the

WILD BEAST

living with everyone who has ever lived!

Thousands of years ago a wild beast came into association with mankind...

The Dog

When the dog gained entrance into people's homes it attempted to domineer them. That is because it was used to living in a pack with an alpha dog that maintained its dominant position by persistent control of the pack. Yapping, snapping and snarling to ensure submission of beta dogs seeking to usurp the canine throne was a common strategy deployed by leaders of these animal packs. Beta dogs realized they could become top dog in a human household quicker and easier than in the home pack. Though humans wised up to dogs pretty quickly, today many dog owners keep their dogs in their homes untrained. To have a life they have to tame the beast to make sure it doesn't take on the role of alpha dog in the family pack.

Cesar Millan, famous as the **Dog Whisperer,** went into homes where dogs had established alpha roles by maintaining dominion over the human family through devious strategies including aggressive behaviour and persistent yapping. Cesar Millan joined the family pack and took over the alpha role from the dog. He used various techniques to gain dominion over the family pet. He then taught the human members of the pack how to maintain control. The premier tool he recommended for training dogs and maintaining control over them was a **collar and lead.**

Cesar Millan said the best way to train a dog is to take it on regular walks with a collar and lead using these to pull it back consistently to heel until it learns to be submissive and do as it is told.

Puppies off the lead rush round out of control. On the lead they constantly pull at it, leaping up or running round in circles. It takes weeks of training ~ pulling them to heel ~ before they settle down, accept you as the boss and behave as you want them to behave.

What on Earth has dog training got to do with alcohol and carbohydrate addiction?

Believe it or not, a lot...

There is the equivalent of a wild beast associated with every one that has to be trained before we can discipline ourselves to fast or abstain from alcohol...

...and I am not referring to the dog, the cat or the pet monkey!

The **wild beast** equivalent of an untamed dog, forever associated with mankind, is

the animal pack psyche in our heads!

THE EGO-MIND

Humans are pack animals and our ego is an animal pack psyche similar to the dog. Unless the dog like psyche is trained, it will take over dominion of our heads as surely as our tail wagging pets will take dominion of our homes. Take the way lap dogs maintain control of people by yapping...

...I challenge you right now to see if you can stop the persistent yakking in your head for even five minutes!

The mind yaks persistently. It is an insidious nagging influence in everyone's head. You may deny this but then denial is a strategy of the controlling psyche that must be confronted to overcome addiction! Alpha dogs depend on the other dogs being weaker than them to maintain control. An individual that is weak is easier to control than an individual that is strong. Alcohol, sugar and other addictive substances weaken us so we are more easily controlled – not by an external conspiracy but by an internal egotistic psyche! Perhaps this accounts for the characteristic denial of the addict - the resistance to any attempt to recognize and overcome the addiction.

Unless we gain control of our ego-minds we will never break habitual addictions because addiction is an aspect of the alpha beta-dog tussle going on in our animal pack psyche!

We each have to deal with a
DOG-OF-A-MIND

Not only is this central to dealing with addiction and securing our health, peace and happiness; it could be absolutely essential for the
SURVIVAL OF OUR SPECIES!

Many pack animals domineer through aggressive behaviour. Aggression is used not only by alpha animals in the pack to maintain control, it is also used by one pack to gain and maintain dominion over another. Packs, tribes, religions, corporations, nations – the name or size of the congregation of animals matters not; the characteristic aggressive behaviour of one pack toward another is the same. One pack of monkeys in Sri Lanka attacking another for territorial dominion was a fascinating feature of a documentary I saw on TV in 2012. The aggression between two primate packs in Sri Lanka over territorial claims, for decades since the 1970's, followed the same characteristic behavioral pattern of primate animal packs; only the Homo sapiens were armed with modern weapons so the consequences were more devastating!

The Israeli-Palestinian conflict is an animal pack struggle for territorial dominion between the tribes of Hebrews and Philistines that has been going on for thousands of years.

Only today, one of the packs is armed with **Nuclear Weapons!**

It is only a matter of time before the primitive primate animal pack psyche leads to their deployment.

In most human relationships one party will use aggressive animal pack strategies in an attempt to control and domineer the other. It is the cause of rows, conflict and war. Unchecked it could lead eventually to a nuclear war and **extinction of our species!**

In *Our Final Century,* top scientist Martin Rees suggests we will not survive the 21st Century. **Desperate times require desperate measures!**

If the **Dog Whisperer** can control the pack-psyche of dogs then maybe we can learn from him how to control the pack-psyche of our own species. Maybe the secret for our survival is for each and every one of us to become a

Mind Whisperer!

The idea is simple. We could apply Cesar Millan's advice for training dogs to the training of our minds. **He suggested we put a collar on the dog, clip on a lead and pull it to heel** until it submits to our will and becomes our servant rather than our master!

I suggest we do the same to our minds.

ARE YOU MAD ASH! HOW CAN YOU PUT A COLLAR & LEAD ON THE MIND?
Actually we are all mad. The only difference between the sane and the insane is the insane chatter away to themselves out loud whereas the sane chatter away to themselves in their heads!

If you want to train your **DOG-OF-A-MIND** you will need a collar and lead...
...and a whistle to call that there **DOG-OF-A-MIND** because it is likely to be chasing random thoughts drifting around in you head!

Believe it or not you have the whistle, collar and lead to train your animal pack psyche built into your body.

IMAGINE; You are just conscious awareness. Your mind is a dog. Its training ground is in your body. A whistle is in your nose, a collar and clip are in your mouth and the lead is in the lungs!

This is how you become a Mind Whisperer
Close your mouth and take three deliberately breaths through your nose. Listen for the sound of your breath in your nasal passages. **Focus on the sound.** This is the whistle to call your DOG-OF-A-MIND from the game it is playing with random passing thoughts.

Bring your attention to the ring of teeth inside of your mouth. That is the collar for your DOG-OF-A-MIND.

Lift up your tongue a few millimeters so the tip is pointing toward the teeth. Do not touch your teeth with your tongue. Just lift it slightly and point it toward the ring of teeth. That is the clip to use to fasten your DOG-OF-A-MIND in its collar. **Taste for a tingling sensation round the tip of your tongue.** That clips the collar to the lead.

The lead for that DOG-OF-A-MIND is your breath. **Bring your attention into your breath.** Breathe slowly and feel the breath go deep into the centre of your lungs. That is how you pull your DOG-OF-A-MIND to heel at your heart. Breathe slow and deep a few times. **Be patient.** Like any technique of mind control it takes practice. Dogs take time to train and your ego-mind will require more persistence and patience to train than a puppy dog.

WALK THE DOG!

Take your DOG-OF-A-MIND on a ten minute walk whenever you can. Go out into nature, to a field or park or into your garden and as you listen for the resonant sound in your nose, lift your tongue slightly pointing it at the collar of teeth to secure your mind in the focus of your attention then breathe slow and deep to bring your DOG-OF-A-MIND to heel in your heart. As you walk, watch each footstep and hold the mind to heel with focused attention on the *feel* of your breath and the *taste* of your tongue pointing at the ring of teeth. Stay aware *simultaneously* of your peaceful deep breathing and the taste of tingling at the tip of your tongue.

Be conscious of the touch of the wind, the sound of birds, the warmth of the sun or cool of the rain and walk on. It doesn't matter how many times that DOG-OF-A-MIND runs off after a thought; the practice is to keep bringing it back to the breath. That is the secret of **MIND WHISPERING.** It's so simple!

An untrained dog is a nightmare.
A trained dog is man's best friend.

An untrained mind is a nightmare.
A trained mind is man's best friend.

START THE PRACTICE

Become a Mind Whisperer NOW!

RELAX WITH THE DOG!

Relax with your DOG-OF-A-MIND. Chill out. Put on gentle, uplifting music. Relax back in a comfortable chair or sofa and practice **Mind Whispering.** Spend twenty minutes to half an hour feeling into your breath. As your DOG-OF-A-MIND settles down with your deep breathing you may begin to feel a power or presence in your heart centre. It may be a subtle sense of well being, a deep feeling of peace or just overall calm and relaxation.

You identify with your body and your mind but, is there more to you? You are aware of thought and are conscious in a body but are you something more fundamental? The constant demands on your attention by your DOG-OF-A-MIND never allow you just to be who you are at the most fundamental level. As you bring your psychic dog under control and have some peace-of-mind you may begin to experience a distinction between yourself and your mind. Discovering yourself is the key to breaking addiction and establishing self discipline. Many people have theories that are not related to direct experience. The ego mind is full of opinions and judgments but if you practice **Mind Whispering** you will experience who you really are and that will help you to be at peace with yourself and find more self control & contentment in your life.

With time and practice you will get into the habit of allowing the consciousness of your tongue and your breath to bring you peace. It will become effortless, especially when relaxed. When your mind is at peace your addictions will have less of a hold on you. In time they may fall away altogether. **BODY CONTROL FOLLOWS MIND CONTROL.**

You can to use **Mind Whispering** to turn away from things and turn your life around in just a few breaths.

Most of us are driven by habit or compulsion. Habitual patterns of thinking and compulsive patterns of behaviour are characteristic of addiction. Freedom is the ability not to think or act by habit or compulsion but to choose to be different, spontaneous and intuitive.

Mind Whispering can help us turn away from alcohol, sugar & junk or fast food. It can help us turn away from an unpleasant thought, an undesirable action, idle gossip, an addictive pattern of behaviour, over-talking, gambling, shop lifting, cheating on a partner etc

The more you practice **Mind Whispering** the easier the practice will become and the easier it will be to fast and abstain from alcohol. It is impossible to discipline the body without first disciplining the mind. If you have a better way than **Mind Whispering;** GO FOR IT!

One act of self discipline will bring more satisfaction than a thousand acts of surrender to addictions.

- ♥ **Mind Whisper** for three breaths then choose to turn away from high calorie food. Feel into the craving with your breath. Remember that most people in the world feel the pangs of hunger. You are not alone.
- ♥ **Mind Whisper** for three breaths then choose to turn away from a tempting drink of alcohol. Feel into the craving with your breath. Remember it is only a few days a week you have to abstain.

Encourage the people close to you to do **Mind Whispering** too so you are not alone in the practice. It is good to have others share your experiences as groups are more successful than individuals in breaking addictions.

You may not succeed every time, especially to begin with. Don't beat yourself up if you fail to turn away from drink or food on a fast day. That is another trick of the DOG-OF-A-MIND to seduce you into giving into addiction then scold you for doing so. If you fail to fast on a fast day, set a new fast day. Just choose another day to practice turning away from food or drink and to practice breaking addictive patterns. Persist. Don't let that DOG-OF-A-MIND get away with its tricks. **Fasting and Mind Whispering work together to provide the healthy discipline necessary to strengthen the will power sufficient to break addictive patterns.** Be patient with yourself. You will eventually succeed if you persist.

PATIENT PERSISTENCE IS THE SECRET OF SUCCESS

Mind Whispering is a very useful and effective tool to help break addictive patterns but there is something else to consider in the battle against addiction...

MALNUTRITION

ALCOHOL AND REFINED CARBOHYDRATES CAN CAUSE MALNUTRITION.

Alcohol Malnutrition

Metabolizing alcohol requires nutrients. As we drink the liver uses up its supply of these nutrients very quickly and they need to be replenished.

The more alcohol we drink the more nutrients we use so more are needed to replace them!

IT'S HARDLY ROCKET SCIENCE!

As we drink more and more alcohol, the blood stream is called upon to replenish the supply of nutrients in the liver from other tissues and organs. As a result, body cells are deprived of critical nutrients and normal body functions suffer.

BE PREPARED FOR COLD TURKEY

If you are a heavy drinker or sugar eater when you start abstaining and fasting you may experience typical withdrawal symptoms including anxiety, irritability, headache, loss of appetite, insomnia, tremors, shakiness, dizziness, depression, impaired cognitive thinking and poor memory; **These will pass!**

Alcohol withdrawal symptoms may be caused by nutrient deficiencies. Vitamin C and the B-complex vitamins are very vulnerable to being destroyed by alcohol. The B vitamins are especially important to mental and emotional well being.

- **Vitamin B_1** (thiamin) deficiencies trigger depression and irritability and can cause neurological and cardiac disorders among alcoholics.

- **Vitamin B$_2$** (riboflavin) deficiency is linked to depression. In 1982 an article published in the *British Journal of Psychiatry* reported that every one of 172 successive patients admitted to a psychiatric hospital for treatment for depression was deficient in B$_2$.

- **Vitamin B$_3$** (niacin) depletion causes anxiety, depression, apprehension and fatigue.

- **Vitamin B$_5$** (pantothenate) symptoms of deficiency are fatigue, chronic stress and depression.

- **Vitamin B$_6$** (pyridoxine) deficiencies can disrupt the formation of neurotransmitters.

- **Vitamin B$_9$** (Folic acid) deficiency is a common cause of depression

- **Vitamin B$_{12}$** (Cyanocobalamin) deficiency will cause depression.

Deficiencies of other nutrients caused by alcohol consumption include A, E, and D along with minerals such as calcium, magnesium and zinc. These can also contribute to the negative feelings that frequently lead susceptible individuals toward another alcoholic beverage.

Increased urine through drinking pints of beer can leach many vital nutrients from the body.

The liver uses an enzyme called **glutathione** to break down toxic substances including alcohol and paracetamol. The amino acids glutamine, glycine and cysteine go to make up glutathione. In the liver alcohol is first changed into toxic acetaldehyde. Then this poisonous substance is turned into harmless acetic acid (vinegar) by glutathione. As glutathione is used up by excess alcohol consumption, acetaldehyde accumulates which can cause symptoms of poisoning such as general malaise, irritability, headache, vomiting and diarrhea. Hangover?

Chronic alcoholics often suffer from malnutrition through poor nutrition resulting from the 'priority' all addicts give to the purchase and consumption of the drug of addiction which often leads to neglect of their overall nutritional welfare.

Alcohol and refined carbohydrates also cause malnutrition through 'empty calories'. Whole grains and pulses, vegetables and fruit, provide a wide variety of nutrients including vitamins, minerals, antioxidants, flavanoids, protein, essential fats, and fibre as well as carbohydrates. Alcohol and refined carbohydrates i.e., white flour and sugar, peeled potatoes and polished rice lack essential nutrients. They provide calories without adequate nutrition. They cheat the body essentially. It feels fed but it is being starved effectively of everything apart from energy ~ except of course for wheat flour which provides the 'gut-glue' protein gluten.

If a poison is described as a substance that harms the body when consumed, alcohol and refined carbohydrates could be described as poisons insofar as they continually spike insulin levels causing, metabolic syndrome the insulin toxicity that predisposes a person to circulatory diseases, cancer, diabetes, obesity, and a host of other degenerative conditions requiring prescribed drugs.

Linked as it is to major causes of death it can safely be said that sugar is poison!

That is not the end of the story. Glucose is actively transported into the body and attracts minerals carrying them in with it. Most minerals are absorbed inefficiently but if they are combined with glucose – calcium as calcium gluconate for example – they are more efficiently absorbed into the body.

When minerals are refined out of carbohydrates the body not only loses them, it loses the opportunity for their efficient absorption. Worse still, the refined glucose in the blood attracts minerals in the blood, making them less available in the body. For example refined glucose will attract calcium from the bones. If we gorge on refined foods such as white bread and sugar, white rice, peeled potatoes, pasta, biscuits, cakes, sweets, sugar drinks, crisps, popcorn, crackers, rice crackers, chocolate, pastries, breakfast cereals... the list is endless...they increase the glucose load in the blood competing with the bones for calcium. No wonder osteoporosis afflicts many people?

Then there is **glucosylation,** the bonding of glucose in the blood to red blood cells and proteins. This 'caramel' like process ~ sugar coating cells ~ sets up chronic disease.

Stupid Question: If vitamins and minerals are refined out of the foods most people eat most of the time where do the majority of people get their vitamins and minerals from?

...And the use of chemical fertilizers, replacing only potassium, phosphorus and nitrogen into the soil, causes fruits, vegetables and grains grown on the soil to become depleted of essential minerals like calcium, magnesium, iron, zinc, chromium, iodine, chromium, boron, manganese, copper, molybdenum, sulphur, zirconium, and selenium... that list is endless too; **and fasting can also deplete us of nutrients.**

Stupid Question: If degenerative diseases are caused by malnutrition and prevention with nutrition costs people money, do they opt for disease rather than health because medical treatment is free and therefore cheaper for them?

After 4 months of fasting two days a week I found that I was beginning to lose too much weight. I am normally skinny but I was beginning to look like an **Oxfam Advert**. So I now fast and feast just one day a week. To reduce the need for strict fasting I developed a green food for my liver, enriched with herbs and fortified with vitamins, minerals and amino acids. I maintain my health with **1 day a week fasting + daily food for the liver ~** with breaks from this too of course. My liver food ensures I am nourished properly when I am feasting, eating supermarket foods and drinking alcohol as well as when I fast. I approached **Indigo Herbs of Glastonbury** and asked them to make my fortified liver food widely available. I now recommend for **EVERYONE especially people who drink even moderate amounts of alcohol regularly** to combine fasting with a liver food containing:

GREEN FOODS:

Barley grass is rich in essential nutrients. Nutritionist, Gillian McKeith, states in her book, "Living Food for Health: 12 Natural Super-foods to Transform Your Health", that barley grass offers more protein than a sirloin steak, five times the amount of iron as broccoli, seven times more vitamin C than orange juice and 11 times more calcium than milk. Barley grass helps to balance the pH of the body. The average Western diet full of processed foods is fairly acidic. Raised acidity in the body is linked to disease and general ill-health. Barley grass is more alkalizing and that helps liver cells to function optimally.

Chlorella is a nutrient-dense super-food that contains 60% protein, 18 amino acids and many essential vitamins and minerals. Chlorella provides the dietary-essential amino acids in excellent ratios. It is also a reliable source of essential fatty acids and contains high levels of chlorophyll, beta-carotene and RNA/DNA. More than 20 vitamins and minerals are found in chlorella, including iron, calcium, zinc, selenium, potassium, magnesium, phosphorous, pro-vitamin A, vitamins C, B1, B2, B2, B5, B6, B12, E and K, biotin, inositol, choline and folate.

ANTIOXIDANTS:

Vitamin C is a powerful antioxidant. My dad, Dr Michael Ash, studied biochemistry at Cambridge under Prof Sir Gowland Hopkins who discovered vitamins. He was in the lab where vitamin C was first isolated. He and the other students were quick to notice that if they took large doses of vitamin C before a party they could stand their drinks and got less hung over which suggests that vitamin C somehow helps of the liver to detox alcohol.

Grape Seed Extract, rich in proanthocyanidin flavonoids, is considered to be one of the most powerful antioxidants known to man ~ especially in combination with Vitamin C. I use them together as they act synergistically ~ small amounts together are more effective than large amounts of either acting alone.

Milk thistle extract nourishes the liver with silymarin flavonoids. I use Milk thistle as it has been known for millennia to benefit the liver.

Turmeric is one of my favourites as it is one of the best natural foods for maintaining a healthy liver. According to the University of Maryland Medical Center website, turmeric has been used for 4,000 years to treat a variety of ailments and is not known to damage the liver, but rather for its protective effects. Turmeric also protects against cancer.

AMINO ACIDS:

I add the amino acids Glutamine, Glycine, & Cysteine as they provide building blocks for the liver detox enzyme **Glutathione.** This is especially useful after a party or visit to a pub.

MINERALS:

Calcium essential for teeth, bones, muscles and a healthy liver is depleted by alcohol and denied by empty calorie foods such as alcohol and refined carbohydrates.

Magnesium is needed for more than 300 biochemical reactions in the body, many occurring in the liver, especially in the regulation of blood sugar levels. Promoting normal blood pressure, magnesium is known to be involved in energy metabolism and there is an increased interest in the role of magnesium in preventing and managing cardiovascular disease, and diabetes.

Zinc is an essential nutrient mineral depleted by alcohol and refined carbohydrates. Zinc is needed for the liver, immune system, and protein synthesis, digestion and control of diabetes, muscle action & semen production.

Selenium is a trace element essential to good health. Vital for the liver it is incorporated into important antioxidant enzymes that help prevent cellular damage from free radicals, regulate thyroid function and support the immune system.

VITAMINS:

B Vitamins: I add all the B Vitamins as they are essential for healthy liver function and especially for metabolizing sugar and alcohol. B vitamin deficiency is linked to chronic alcoholism and metabolic syndrome.

Vitamin D I add as it is essential for liver health, calcium uptake and is sorely lacking in many people in Britain today.

Vitamin E from the diet and supplements ~ may lower the risk of liver cancer. (*J. Nat. Cancer Institute* July 17 2012).

Vitamin A is important but good diets contain sufficient and excess can damage the liver.

Iron is an essential mineral but too much can harm the liver. It is abundant in good diets. Consult your doctor for an anemia check if you think you need additional iron.

FOODS TO HELP THE LIVER

Garlic contains numerous compounds that activate the liver enzymes responsible for flushing out toxins. Garlic also contains allicin and selenium, two powerful nutrients proven to help protect the liver from toxic damage, and aid it in the detoxification process.

Grapefruit - rich in natural vitamin C (when fresh) and antioxidants - is a powerful liver cleanser containing compounds that increase the production of liver detox enzymes and the flavonoid *naringenin* that encourages the liver to burn fat rather than store it.

Green Tea contains catechins, natural plant antioxidants that help eliminate accumulated liver fat and promote proper liver function Green tea also helps protect the liver against toxins that can cause liver damage.

Green leafy vegetables including fresh celery, leeks, chives and spring onions, water cress and rocket, bitter gourd, dandelion greens, spinach, mustard greens and chicory are good foods for the liver as they contain cleansing compounds which help eliminate pollutants.

Apricots are low in calories but rich in antioxidants, fiber, vitamins, and minerals. They contain numerous liver loving phytochemicals and zeaxanthin: good for the eyes.

Avocados, rich in glutathione-producing compounds, promote liver health by helping it repair itself, protect against toxic overload, and encourage its cleansing ability.

Walnuts, which contain high levels of the amino acid l-arginine, glutathione, and omega-3 fatty acids, help detoxify the liver of disease-causing ammonia. Extracts from their hulls are used for liver-cleansing.

REGULAR FASTING COUPLED WITH GOOD NUTRITION CAN HELP THE BODY DEAL WITH SUGAR AND THE LIVER ALSO REQUIRES SPECIAL NUTRITION TO HELP IT COPE WITH ALCOHOL HOWEVER LEGISLATION IS NEEDED <u>URGENTLY</u> TO CONTROL THE MARKETING OF THESE DANGEROUS DRUGS.

ANGER

A compromised liver is related to anxiety & anger

Anxiety and anger are commonplace today in the general population where alcohol and carbohydrate addiction are normal and chemicals pollute the body. Aggression and irritability are common side effects of the deadly drug alcohol resulting in widespread anti-social behaviour, crime, abuse, domestic rows and breakdown in relationships.

A TOXIC LIVER CAN LEAD TO A TOXIC MIND

We can counteract anger & hatred with gratitude and love.

WATER

Drink lots of water after alcohol to flush the liver

Some scientists believe that water has memory from its *molecular structure* which can influence health or disease. (*Water the Great Mystery* 2006) They claim to have shown in experiments that water is affected by the mind and that thoughts of love and gratitude are more beneficial than hate & anger. Whereas skeptics treat this research with derision, if you are more open minded you might like to use water to send messages of love to your liver ~ before drinking water speak over it:

"Thank you, I love you!"

Stupid Question: Why are skeptics so offended by people who believe there is more to life than they do?

FOOD ADDICTION

Sugar Speed

The speed sucrose and starch are digested into sugar (glucose) and absorbed is called **Glycemic Index (GI)**

Sugar Load

How much a food eaten raises blood glucose levels is its **Glycemic Load**

Fasting reduces the sugar load

Healthy Eating reduces the sugar speed

Sugar Speed is like *Volts in electricity* it gives the body a *Sugar Shock* and the faster the speed the greater the shock!

The body reacts to **Sugar Shock &
Sugar Load** by releasing **INSULIN**
which leads to deposition of fat in the
belly and cholesterol in arteries:

Sugar Shock
= Fat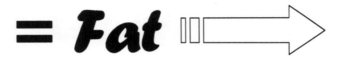

> ➢ **Obesity**
> ➢ **Heart Disease**
> ➢ **Stroke**

&Insulin Resistance type II

> ➢ **Diabetes**

Cooking starch swells it so it is digested into sugar and absorbed faster therefore cooking increases *sugar shock*

Cooked Food ⟹ Disease

Raw Food decreases *sugar shock*

Raw Food ⟹ Health

FIBRE slows down the digestion of starch into sugar and its absorption so

Fibre decreases *sugar shock*

Natural High Fibre Whole Food ⟹ Health

Raw Food ⟹ High Fibre Healthy

Food Processing cooks food and refines fibre out of it so

Processed Food ⟹ Disease

Processed Food = *Sugar Shock* which drops blood sugar levels, making you hungry so you buy and eat more sugary processed food which causes more **SUGAR SHOCKS** so more insulin is released, driving more sugar to fat causing you put on more weight.

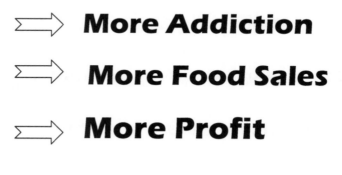

⟹ **More Addiction**

⟹ **More Food Sales**

⟹ **More Profit**

⟹ *More Disease*

Processed foods make us unhealthy for profit and Pharmaceutical drugs then profit from our ill health

REMEMBER THE DRUG BARONS

They make money from the deadly cycle of addiction, disease and death!

Check out the BBC 1 Brian Cox documentary Addicted To Pleasure 26th Nov 2012, 9pm

Processed food, sugary food & take away Fast Foods are zero rated for VAT & like alcohol are advertised & are on tempting display in shops cafes and supermarkets, yet these addictive substances cause as much disease and death as tobacco...

and what about children?

CHILDREN

We are concerned to protect children from becoming drug and tobacco addicts but we

Encourage them to eat sugar and Fast Food from an early age when

FAST FOODS & SUGAR ARE HIGHLY ADDICTIVE LIKE ALCOHOL, DRUGS AND TOBACCO

The fashion of relying on Fast Food is driving the obesity epidemic, especially in children.

We need to fast Not eat Fast Food

Food is known to be addictive:

Food and Addiction: A Comprehensive Handbook (Oxford University Press 2012)

This first book compiling academic essays describes the science behind food addiction and claims food can be as addictive as drugs, cigarettes and alcohol... The primary editors of this book, Kelly Brownell, Professor of public health at Yale and Mark Gold, addiction expert and Professor at the University of Florida, College of Medicine, emphasize the seriousness of food addiction and link it to the global epidemic of obesity. They stress the need to look at food, drugs, alcohol & tobacco in the same way, i.e. as highly addictive substances that can cause disease.

IF TOP SCIENTISTS ARE CALLING FOR ADDICTIVE FOOD, ALCOHOL, DRUGS AND TOBACCO TO BE TREATED THE SAME...

...WHY AREN'T THEY TREATED THE SAME IN LAW?

WHERE IS THE FAIRNESS IN THE LAW?

Until alcohol and addictive foods are treated in law like TOBACCO

THE LAW IS AN ASS

My father Dr Michael Ash was the first medical doctor to declare openly the link between cigarette smoking and lung cancer in the 1950's. Since then the law has restricted the promotion and sale of tobacco products. Sixty years on I am calling for all foods that cause disease, alcohol and drugs to be treated in law like tobacco because tobacco legislation and health warnings have been effective in reducing the numbers smoking.

LIKE TOBACCO
DISEASE CAUSING FOOD PRODUCTS AND ALCOHOL COULD

➢ Be banned from advertising
➢ Carry health warnings
➢ Be banned from open display in shops and supermarkets
➢ Be sold behind counters
➢ Be banned from using logos and colourful packaging
➢ Be restricted in availability to children and adolescents
➢ Display pictures of death and disease on labels and packs ~ as depicted on cigarette packs
➢ Be restricted in public places; alcohol already is because of antisocial behaviour but also addictive foods because of...

PASSIVE SUGAR SHOCK

Just like passive smoking, people don't have to even eat addictive food to get disease. People can suffer a release of insulin by just the sight, smell, or reminder of food.

The only macro food that doesn't cause this ***sugar shock effect*** is

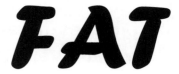

FAT is the only food that doesn't cause passive fattening!

The Research: "High acute
levels of insulin can be produced simply by seeing and thinking about food and individuals showing this response show a greater tendency toward weight gain in a food abundant environment...elevations in insulin produce increased hunger, heightened perceived pleasantness of sweet taste and increased food intake." (Judith Rodin, *Health Psychology,* Vol. 4(1) 1985, 1-24)

"Stimulants for insulin secretion can range from seeing, smelling or tasting food to increases in food molecules in the blood."
(www.healio.com/endocrinology/news June 5, 2012)

On June 25, 2012 Dr Kathleen Page of the University of Southern California, Keck School of Medicine (Los Angeles) read a paper at the US Endocrine Society 94th Annual Meeting at Houston Texas revealing that in the brains of obese women when they looked at sugary food the centers, related to laying down fat lit up.

Chocolate does not contain addictive substances but it is addictive because the sight, smell or taste of it lights up the addictive centers in the brain.

Stupid Question: How come governments have done nothing to restrict addictive food displays when the harm they cause was known way back in 1985?

The deliberate display of food to make you hungry so you crave and buy more food is

CONSUMER ABUSE

Walking down the street you can be confronted by displays of delicious food in shop windows or smells of baking bread, sizzling bacon or yummy frying doughnuts. At no fault of your own insulin is secreted, glucose is taken out of your blood and converted into glycogen and fat and you are left craving for food because of the drop in your blood sugar. This abuse of your blood sugar levels makes it hard for you not to buy the tempting food. If you are overweight or diabetic, food displays and smells exacerbate your disease. **That is an abuse of consumers.** At home you can be abused by pictures of pizza or chocolates pushed through you letter box and adverts for foods on your TV screens.

> **CONSUMER ABUSE** can cause people to gain weight.
> **CONSUMER ABUSE** can make it difficult to fast or diet.
> **CONSUMER ABUSE** can exacerbate serious diseases.

...You have a right to queue to pay for your fuel without being subjected to consumer abuse!

Insulin secretions induced by the shelves of chocolate lining kiosk aisles can cause a drop in blood sugar of waiting customers so they crave for chocolate and find it hard not to buy a bar or two. **Even if they DO NOT buy the chocolate bars CUSTOMERS can still suffer WEIGHT GAIN & increase INSULIN resistence leading to obesity and diabetes.**

IN PRACTICALLY EVERY FUEL STATION WHEN WE QUEUE TO PAY WE ARE EXPOSED TO THIS FORM OF CONSUMER ABUSE

THINK ABOUT IT!

- There is an epidemic of obesity and diabetes.
- Disease is caused not just by eating addictive foods but by the sight or smell of them.
- We have a right to go about our business without being constantly tempted to consume addictive foods.
- All addictive substances should be controlled by the same laws. That is common sense. Anything else is unfair practice, discrimination and a miscarriage of justice.
- But treating food and alcohol as class A drugs would be madness and impossible.

The Criminal Drug Laws Don't Work. Criminalizing Drugs Creates Crime.

Prohibition of alcohol in America did not work. It created crime.

Prohibition of drugs today does not work. It simply creates crime.

AND HEALTH AND SAFETY LAWS ARE SHEER HYPOCRISY WHILE THE LAW PERMITS THE DISPLAY AND PROMOTION OF ADDICTIVE SUBSTANCES THAT CAUSE MORE DISEASE & DEATH THAT CLASS A DRUGS!

THERE IS A CASE FOR ADDICTIVE FOODS TO BE TREATED IN LAW LIKE MEDICAL DRUGS BECAUSE THEY DO MODIFY HUMAN PHYSIOLOGY IN A WAY THAT CAUSES DISEASE!

...Insulin so essential to life for the control of blood sugar is turned into a disease causing **TOXIN** by many foods.

As well as toxic levels of insulin the liver has to cope with a host of toxins from the environment produced by the **CHEMICAL INDUSTRY.**

Since World War II:

- 75,000 man made chemicals released into the environment
- 5,000 of them cause cancer
- 250 are in your fat cells **NOW**
- Prescribed drugs from the toilet pollute the environment where many of them are active
- Antibiotic overuse has led to antibiotic resistant **super-bugs**

The Liver must detox all these deadly products of the chemical Industry

How can the liver detox effectively if it is overburdened with addictive food and alcohol, clogged with fat and overwhelmed with insulin?

No wonder cancer is the #2 cause of death?

How can we save ourselves?

What hope is there for our children confronted with a future of debt and disease?

What hope is there for our children to live long, happy and healthy lives free of debt and disease?

How can we live a Healthy Life?

HEALTHY LIVING

Healthy Eating + Fresh Air + Exercise + Pure Water is the formula for **Healthy Living**

EXERCISE BURNS CALORIES

OXYGEN BURNS CALORIES

EXERCISE + OXYGEN + WATER

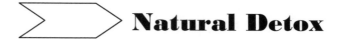 **Natural Detox**

Living on the land provides **Exercise + Water + Fresh Air + Fresh Whole Natural Food**

If only more people had the opportunity to move onto a few acres for a healthy lifestyle for themselves and their children...

...where they could be
- ➢ Less exposed to addictive foods
- ➢ Less exposed to alcohol
- ➢ Less exposed to drugs
- ➢ Less exposed to toxic chemicals
- ➢ More exposed to nature
- ➢ More likely to eat healthy food
- ➢ More likely to exercise frequently
- ➢ More exposed to fresh air

Is it possible for people to

RETURN to THE LAND?

We can return to the land in towns and cities through urban gardens and allotments but not to a full time, rural, self-sustained lifestyle unless we can buy a farm but farms have too much land & are costly.

WHAT IS THE REALISTIC OPPORTUNITY TO LIVE WHERE WE GROW OUR OWN FOOD?

We can grow food in an urban garden, an allotment or on a farm if we own one but...

We are not allowed to live on agricultural land; land where food is grown.

A tragic item I saw on TV in 2012 was the eviction of a young couple from their own land where they were settled with their children in a temporary home. They were living sustainably & debt free, growing their own vegetables with a compost toilet & chickens. Then, the council forced them off their land and they had to return to non sustainable, urban living.

Stupid Question: How can people live sustainably in the country if they have to hold down a job to pay rent and bills on a house in town?

The rural population left the land for industry but the urban population can't leave industry and return to the land!
There are people who would choose the healthy lifestyle of living and working on the land, to grow their own food, build their own homes, rear their families in a healthy natural rural environment with fresh air, exercise and a minimal carbon footprint, without debt or state benefit if they could but

PLANNING WILL NOT ALLOW!

THE PLANNING LAWS KEEP US IN TOWNS AND CITIES WHERE WE ARE EXPOSED CONTINUALLY TO

CONSUMER ABUSE

In town & city, where there are shops, fuel stations, restaurants, shopping malls, & supermarkets we are more exposed to alcohol & addictive foods than in the country.

Especially in supermarkets we are encouraged, with loaded shelves of tempting displays, shopping trolleys, gaudy packaging and discounted prices, to consume sugar and alcohol, the continuous over consumption of which are connected to stroke and heart disease, cancer, diabetes, Alzheimer's disease, liver disease and the need for prescribed drugs.

In the urban environment we are exposed to consumerism in a supermarket and fast food culture that fosters degenerative disease.

In the urban environment our children are brought up as consumers in the supermarket and fast food culture that fosters degenerative disease.

Action is needed NOW

It is a matter of life and death that all drugs and addictive substances are dealt with effectively; that people are allowed to choose healthy lifestyles and the exposure to all forms of abuse is curtailed.

Imagine a dreadful storm. A bridge is washed away. You know your friends are driving toward the bridge unaware of the danger they are in. Would you just get on with your own thing or would you to get on your mobile and warn them before it is too late? More people suffer misery, disease and slow death through easily preventable degenerative diseases than through car accidents or any other cause of sickness and death so...

IF you love your friends and family, pass this book onto them to warn them of the danger they are in before it is too late! Let's work together to make a difference in this world. If you are concerned about drugs, food addiction and consumer abuse, give a copy of this book ~ available from Amazon ~ to your doctor, solicitor, MP and MEP.

THE LEGACY
© Leticia Parmer

How cheerfully we sew the seeds of our demise,
How happily we'll eat another bacon slice,
How innocently on our skin the cooking sunshine lies,
How unaware the passengers,
Showering benzene from the skies,
No one thinks of death at times like these,
And yet it's then we silently sew the seeds,
Of that most virulent disease,
We neither see nor feel the cell mutate,
To slowly, silently create,
A chemistical change that seals our fate,
And then....it simply is too late,
Yet, it is in our hands, it's our choice,
Can you, one person, one small voice,
Open the eyes and hearts of man,
To know he kills himself .... You can!

If the lies had not occurred,
If governments had kept their word,
If theft of land, of ritual and rite,
Had not transpired, why then, there might,
Have been a different human history,
Of health, instead of tragedy,
Tobacco, sacred once, now kills,
Where native spirits blessed the hills,
And sugar, wrenched from slaving brow,
Creates an epidemic now,
Of death through fatness, sloth and greed,
Let's take no more than we truly need.

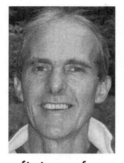 I was born in Kent in 1948 graduated in nutrition at Queen Elizabeth College London University in 1972. In the field of nutrition my main interest was mineral malnutrition caused by the refining of sugar. I then became concerned about migraine and taught sufferers how to control their affliction with diet. I had a break from nutrition for a number of years to devote myself to my other life-long interest, physics. My latest book: *Vortex of Energy* (PujaPowerPublications 2012 £12.50) is an easy-to-understand, refreshing alternative to quantum mechanics. In 2010 my concern for nutrition and health was rekindled when my nephew, Bruce, called on me to reconsider my father's work on vitamins and alcohol. My focus is now on the liver, and the extent this vital organ is abused by food and drink. Currently I am cooperating with **INDIGO HERBS** of Glastonbury to develop green food products for those who share my concern for the liver and wish to use nutrition as a means of maintaining health without compromised lifestyles.